AF211927

M.D. READY

HEALTHY GUY

**The Ultimate Guide Towards a Happier and Healthier You,
Learn All the Useful Information and Tips on How You
Can Shape Up and Have a Better Life**

Descrierea CIP a Bibliotecii Naţionale a României
M.D. READY
    HEALTHY GUY. The Ultimate Guide Towards a Happier and Healthier You, Learn All the Useful Information and Tips on How You Can Shape Up and Have a Better Life / M.D. Ready – Bucharest: Editura My Ebook, 2020
    ISBN

M.D. READY

HEALTHY GUY

**The Ultimate Guide Towards a Happier and Healthier You,
Learn All the Useful Information and Tips on How You
Can Shape Up and Have a Better Life**

My Ebook Publishing House
Bucharest, 2020

TABLE OF CONTENTS

FOREWORD

Day in day out we keep ourselves absorbed with those things that matter the most to us. A lot of times, it might be just to survive and make a living. In doing so we from time to time disregard or forget about the extra matters that are necessary to balance our lives. They're even more crucial to provide real meaning to our world.

You have to pay attention to your health.

Exercise is where it's at, along with a low-fat, high-fiber diet and a wish to move toward good health. Naturally you'll likewise need to cut back on those awful habits, like smoking, drinking excessively, or drug use, which includes over usage of prescription drugs.

There's no magic bullet that will make you lose weight without trying. No particular diet that lets you eat a ton of food and drop pounds quick. No ab-machine or exercise bike that you see in the middle of the night on an infomercial is truly going to make that much difference to you.

We all know the secret to slimming down, right? Eat right, exercise more and keep a positive attitude. Yes, we all know that.

If you ever had a weight issue though, you know it's not really that easy. Eating right is difficult when you're facing steady hunger, when every food that's good for you tastes awful and you're racing full speed ahead from the minute you wake up till you hop into bed at night making fast food truly tempting. Exercise is time consuming and hard, at times it could even be downright terrible! As for that favorable attitude, well that's relatively easy. Once you get past the hunger pangs and the sore muscles, the fact that you have not eaten anything that you like in a week and a half and have worn blisters, in places better not mentioned, on that bike seat.

After that staying positive is a piece of cake. Well, no, I guess it truly isn't.

Good health comes to those that attend to their Body. When you better your health today health, in turn additional good things will come to you in a lot of ways. Before you know it you'll discover yourself doing things you never did before.

While only the higher power is in control of our earthly life, it doesn't mean we can't attempt to live a healthy and happy life. In attending to our bodies, and having a complimentary life-style, we will live longer…

Do you wish to live longer, happier, and healthier? If you truly wish to, reading this e-Book can help you achieve your goals........

Get all the info you need here.

Healthy Happy You

Everything You Need To Know To Shape Up And
Have A Better Life

CHAPTER 1

THE BASICS

Synopsis

The following are some considerations that should be look and get you started with the basics.

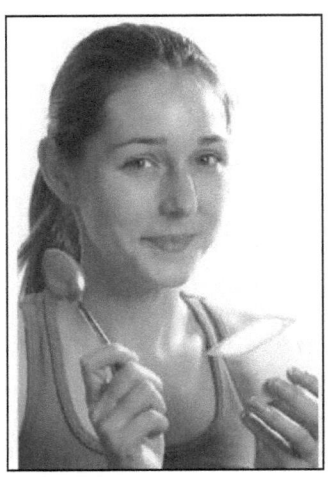

The Basics

- Rest will help with body functions and help you have less stress, and anxiety.

Sleep helps you to think clearly. Get a sound routine for rest. Discover how much sleep you really need. During the day if you're not working, take a 30 minute nap, which might help you feel better during the evening. Everyone is different so you'll have to see what amount of sleep your body requires.

- Nutrition, vitamins and the right food will help you to live the life you'd like to live.

The body needs nutrients to function, and without a suitable diet we'll be starving vital organs and they won't function correctly. Gluttony isn't great for the body either and makes the heart work harder.

Left out of the eat-less-and-exercise- more truism, is the fact that we're not only physical beings but spiritual ones as well.

However, action needs to be taken. Individuals are gaining weight at an alarming rate. From our eldest persons to our youngest, we're plumping up at levels never seen previously.

A few physicians and other health care providers claim eating food that's healthy for you is more crucial than exercising. However is it true?

- Exercise on a day-to-day bases will step-up the chances of not getting brittle bones and stiff joints when you get older.

Exercising will better your pulse, which will ensure a healthier life-style and keep you from feeling sluggish. Stress and anxiety may be cut down with exercising. If you're not doing any exercise, begin today. Don't get into huge workouts to begin with. Do easy arm lifts, leg lifts, even simply stretching. Walk up and down stairs, if you're able to utilize stairs, at a slow pace a few times daily. After a week you are able to introduce your body to a bit more exercise. Take your time.

- We have to address 3 main areas if we wish to bring about long-run weight-loss: the mental, emotional and physiological facets.

This will be a road even as hard as the strictest diet and as painful as running a marathon. It might be, but it's not. Using a couple of simple strategies, you're able to bolster your self-control, your metabolic rate and your favorable feelings about losing weight. You're able to likewise relieve hunger pains and feelings of angst over your present weight.

You're able to do this yourself, or have a acquaintance or professional help you with them, so don't be concerned that you might not have ever tried anything like this before!

Here are a few basic techniques you're able to utilize to aid in losing weight. While simple they're truly powerful. You still have to diet and exercise; these strategies will make that easier to do though.

Begin by calming yourself and quieting your mind. Just take a moment to not worry about anything, relax and let go of any distractions.

Think in your mind that you're already slim. I know that this feels unusual, but if you wish to lose weight it helps to convince yourself that it's possible. If your brain rebels and tries to tell you something different merely replace the thought with the idea you're thin and healthy and don't fret about it. It will take a bit of time to train your subconscious how to be slender.

Spend a few minutes simply "knowing" that you're slim and trim. You don't even have to picture it. As a matter of fact, to your deeper self it's more helpful if you don't picture it.

Now imagine your day. "See" yourself consuming a healthy breakfast. Do what you need to till lunch. Think about all this time passing without a great deal of hunger. Envisage enjoying a lunch of healthy foods that you organized in the morning.

Know that errors will occur and you'll let them go. See yourself doing some exercise and truly enjoying it, is it hard? Certainly, but nothing you can't handle! Run through dinner in this way as well. Notice that you're not craving sweets in particular; hunger isn't an issue for you either. Perhaps you'll have a small snack before bed? That's up to you.

The crucial thing here is to utilize conceptual thought as much as conceivable. If you haven't gotten the trick of thinking in ideas as yet, simply do your best.

- Water will help your body to do away with toxins, germs and things that your body doesn't need.

Water is the sole fluid that will truly flush your system out. It's extremely suggested that you drink adequate water every day. Remember next time you have to buy something to drink, get a bottle of water. You'll save cash and your health will benefit without the sugar and additional ingredients in a soda pop.

- Protect yourself from harm.

Do you like to ride a bicycle? Put on a helmet. Don't say ah that's not for me. Youngsters and grownups are hurt everyday with bicycle accidents. Protect your head, and your brain.

- Use good moisturizers and lotions to protect the skin from too much sun.

Lotions and moisturizers will help keep skin healthy. As we mature the skin will start to break down and thin. Utilizing good lotion and moisturizers will help your body to keep your skin in the correct shape.

- Stress, depression and tension need to be cut down in an individual's life.

Not only is it harmful to your emotional state, it's causing stress to the heart. We have to control these matters and learn to unwind.

- You must lay off Smoking.

Not too much more to say about that. It isn't good, smells foul, and tastes foul. Your heart and lungs don't enjoy it either. Give it up.

- Observe the doctor appointments.

See your doctor as frequently as they'd like you to go. Have annual checkups to ensure that things are all right with you. We have to take an attack of preventive care.

CHAPTER 2

IN DEPTH CONCEPTS

Synopsis

If you wish happiness you have to reach within, rely on your natural instincts and let them guide you. If you wish to live longer and healthier you have to conform to a healthy lifestyle, which is exempt of drugs, chemicals, substances, particular habits, behavior, and so on. You have to work out to better the metabolic process, bones, joints, and muscles.

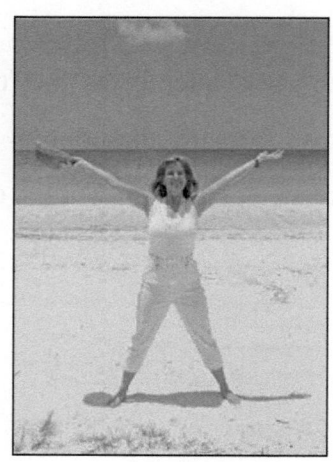

Next we're going to look at several separate concepts in a row. These will in reality be building powerful spiritual fields around you, so make sure you keep the ideas/concepts you're maintaining really clear and as constant as conceivable.

Looking Deeper

As humans we have to have spiritual, mental, and physical nutrients to keep us fit and strong. Spiritual nutrients includes prayer, a deeper comprehending of the truths from the higher power, and ongoing cleanliness of the mind and body. The body is our temple and if we use substances, eat or drink bad junk, like too much alcohol or engage in injurious actions we'll suffer misery, pitiful health, and our life will shorten.

A few of the things we do in life might cause us harm. If we don't get proper rest it might over time induce heart issues, as well as additional health worries. You have to stop bad habits and start fresh health patterns to move towards living healthier. Most people fail to see that the way they conduct themselves might cause stress, which makes them distressed.

The beginning of each health plan is eating correctly, exercise and acquiring proper rest. If you stick with healthy foods with the proper vitamins and supplements you'll be able to get to a healthier life. One of the .main issues today is that unhealthy ingredients are put into our food that's touching the lives of millions. Among the reasons that obesity is increasing is due to things added to foods, which cause weight gain and cravings.

Many people listen to what they wish to hear and brush off what they wish to avoid. Occasionally we have to look at the facts. If you're drinking excessively and your friends or loved ones tell you about it, hear what they're saying as you're not only hurting yourself, you're likewise hurting the people you love.

Emotional reaction might turn into a damaging reaction, which might make an individual distressed. If an person is distressed, it lessens life span, as well as wellness.

Learning to reword things might help to better communications with others. Frequently relationships fall apart if inactive listening happens. For instance, if somebody is upset they may strike out at somebody emotionally, he in turn reacts negatively. This all leads to sadness and will cause ill health, successively shortening your life.

Surely we all daydream or skip out for a moment, yet if we take it too far and utilize it as an attempt to escape truth, we're only causing harm. If you wish to be happier you'll have to get a grip on this kind of conduct and/or habit.

A different big issue is judging. Scores of people judge and rarely do they sincerely get to know the person they judge. If you wish to live a happier life, quit judging others. If you don't wish to be judged, quit judging others. Bear in mind... Judge others as you wish them to judge you.

You've choices between good and bad. If you're seeking the good in someone, you'll most likely discover it. If you're seeking the bad in someone you'll most likely discover it. The choice is yours. Regrettably, from time to time it so happens that the bad takes charge in people's lives, crushing the good in them.

Many people think they read minds. They frequently put words in the mouth of others, instead of hearing what is really said to them. Don't do it.

Next are some specific drills to go through for a healthier and slimmer body:

Carry the thought of energy in your body. Feel the energy flowing through you. Buzzing and exciting your system. This will step-up your metabolic rate. Feel it in every part of your body. Hold this for at least a minute.

Hold the thought of warmth. Beginning in the center of your body and warming each part of your being. This will step-up your metabolism even more. Once again maintain for at least a minute.

Carry the idea of a lack of hunger. This is so powerful that you must utilize care not to strip yourself of hunger all together. This will in reality dampen your sense of physical hunger and appetite. Continue this for a minute.

At last, hold the concept of happiness. Everyone ought to practice this irrespective of their want to lose pounds! It will build up your morale enough to stick with your diet and exercise program.

There are a lot of additional things that can be done to help a person slim down using spiritual techniques. For instance pain control techniques might make exercise more pleasant, as might simple mood elevation.

Ideas of what sorts of foods are tasty might be altered both internally and externally of yourself with a little help. Metabolism might be increased and body might be triggered to expel fat rather than conserve it.

Certainly, you'll still have to watch what you eat.

Yes, physical activity is great for you and should be part of your daily program. These and additional spiritual healing techniques might help to increase the ease and effectiveness of weight loss efforts though, making a definite gain in your quality of life.

If you would like to try these strategies but fear you don't have the skill level needed, try and enlist an acquaintance to give you a hand.

If that isn't a choice you might try getting professional help to make things simpler in the short-term. With practice though, you're able to learn to do all of these things and more on your own. That you have the power to control these things is clear.

Now the question is, do you decide to take charge of your weight, or do you keep doing what you have always done?

It's up to you.

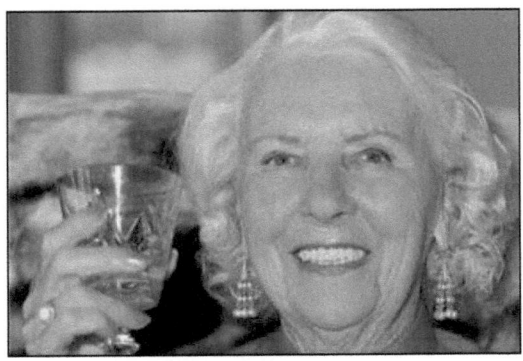

CHAPTER 3

BE HAPPIER

Synopsis

We all have days if the world appears to fall on our shoulders. At these times we could feel living healthier, longer, and happier is out of reach. A few of us deal with tension as it comes our way, while others find it hard to handle.

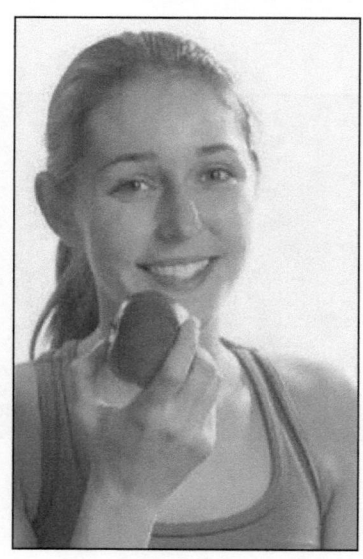

Behaviors, thinking formulas, habits, conduct, and the like calls for adjusting to live a happier life. If you let awful behaviors dominate your brain, you're injuring your health.

A Better Way Of Life

If you paraphrase during communication you summarize what is being said. If you reiterate info it clears up communication, which develops a much richer relationship. Let's view an illustration to help you see how paraphrasing might reduce argument, relieving tension and leading to better health as well as helping with stress eating.

Sue: John, I need to buy a new dress for the upcoming event. John:You want a new dress?

Sue: Well, yes, I'd enjoy a new dress.

John: You're stating you wish to buy a new dress for the approaching event. So, are you asking me if it's all right to buy the dress? (Clarifying)

Sue: Yes dear,

John: I'm fine with that. If you want a new dress, buy one.
Sue: Thanks.

This is an simple paraphrase, yet you are able to see how it clears up the conversation. Paraphrasing will arrest passive listening. It will likewise rectify any allegations, assumptions, or misconstrued communication. If you paraphrase you likewise make one another happy, since you'll feel heard and noticed. Communication works both ways and if you paraphrase you are able to cut down angry emotions, which frequently escalate if info is misconstrued. It's a good way to better memory as well. If emotions are tumultuousness it bears on the heart, which frequently leads to mediocre health. If you wish to live happier, you have to control your emotions. Clarifying is a way to command emotions.

Negativity will only lead to ill health and breakdown in relationships. It leads to sorrow and pessimistic thinking. Basically, negative energy (emotions) is self-denial. It's a vast problem that's causing individuals to suffer. A few of the consequences of damaging energy (emotional response) are coronary failure, hypertension, strokes, heart attacks and so forth.

An person with positive energy will reflect on others, and frequently the energy will spread warmth. If you learn to formulate positive energy you'll glitter like a star, which will make you feel pleased inside.

What is the issue? Tension is a daily factor that we all have to face. There's no way around stress. If you discover how to minimize stressors and bring down tension it might make your life easier. Among the best ways to bring down stress is performing stretching exercises. With this in mind we can give a few helpful tips to teach you to reduce stress. When you do regular workouts, you're working to boost energy, rest sounder, boost self-respect, etc.

Tension is the leading cause of assorted sicknesses, and today stress is becoming among the biggest killers in the world. The first thing you have to be cognizant of is the signs of tension. Recognizing the signs might help you fight back, and win the battle.

If you feel edgy, jittery, or restlessness is taking charge, most likely you're stressed. Sensitivity, pessimistic thinking, and taking offense to what other people say to you are signs of tension.

If you're jerking nervously, biting your nails, pulling hair, or wiggling the knees you likely are feeling tension. Nausea, irregularity, diarrhea, excessive smoking, depending on alcohol or drugs are all signs of tension. If you begin to feel cranky frequently and your patience is thin, you're walking around strained. Frequently the irritability moves to uptight feelings, stress, and belligerent or obsessive-compulsive behaviors.

When you forget frequently, discover it hard to concentrate, your brain is overwhelmed with thoughts, feel disconnected, are not able to think distinctly you're most likely stressed. Tiredness and overwhelming feelings of pressure are signs. As well, it might include, low self-respect, anxiety, panic attacks, anger, bitterness, crying for nothing, moodiness, nightmares, and inability to express joy.

If you feel stressed, you may experience tension of the muscles and tiredness. You'll likely experience back, head, shoulder, and neck pain. Your eyes may feel tired and the muscles might twitch, particularly around the corners of your eyes. Frequently the jaw feels stiff, while the mouth feels dry. The palms of the hands might feel sweaty, while the fingers will feel cold. You may experience heartburn and indigestion frequently, as well as bladder and urinary problems. You may also experience trembling of the heart, weight gain or loss, headaches, colds, hyperventilation, and so forth.

Among the ways to cut back stress is to comprehend the principals of eating a balanced diet. Curbing stress is crucial. It's crucial to eat 3 balanced meals daily, or spread the meals out to 5 little portions daily. If eating you ought to avoid eating
28

quickly, preferably take your time and let the food process in the digestive system. Include 5 helpings of fruits and veggies in your daily plan. Drinking a glass of water one-half an hour before and after meals may help you maintain weight.

Regular work outs will help you unwind, rest well, raise your energy while raising your self-regard and confidence. You'll look and feel great. A general schedule should include daily activities for twenty to thirty minutes. If you've issues getting moving, begin slowly and gradually work into a full routine.

Posture is crucial. Before you start a workout always check your posture, which ought to be aligned. Keeping it straight might help you avoid bone related disease and encourage better breathing, which relieves tension. It will further relaxation, better confidence, as well as make you appear younger, in shape, and slimmer. It will also raise energy and vitality, which is crucial.

Try to turn in at the same time every night. Sleep will bring down tension. Modify your bedroom if you find it difficult to sleep. A change might make you feel more relaxed. Keep the room dark and hushed when you're sleeping. Make sure that your mattress and pillow fits your posture and makes you feel relaxed. Don't use caffeine, smoke, or drink before retiring.

You're able to work out an hour before bedtime to get tired. If you frequently awaken during the night and discover it difficult to sleep, get out of bed and read a book.

Train your brain to think only during wake hours, to unwind and think positive. Attempt to focus on one task at a time, which will encourage memory and relaxation. Try not to fret, rather do something about it.

Your attitude plays a huge part. When you've a favorable outlook or attitude it moves you to achieve your goals and plans.

Stretching exercises and meditation call for proper breathing. Breathe naturally while exercising, meditating etc. Get aware of your breathing and practice breathing properly. This will help you relax.

Stretching might help to flex the joints, which encourages solid muscles. Stretching will open the air passages, and help you to feel relaxed.

Before starting exercise you may wish to use meditation. Meditation helps to clear your mind and implement positive thinking. You have to practice centering your attention while doing meditation. Some people want to listen to soft sounds, while others center better on objects. Mediation is enlightenment of the spiritual mind. When you meditate correctly you practice straight posture, breathing, centering, and attitude. Practicing

30

meditation will promote awareness, as well as encourage relaxation. If the mind and body loosens up, it boosts health, life span, and happiness.

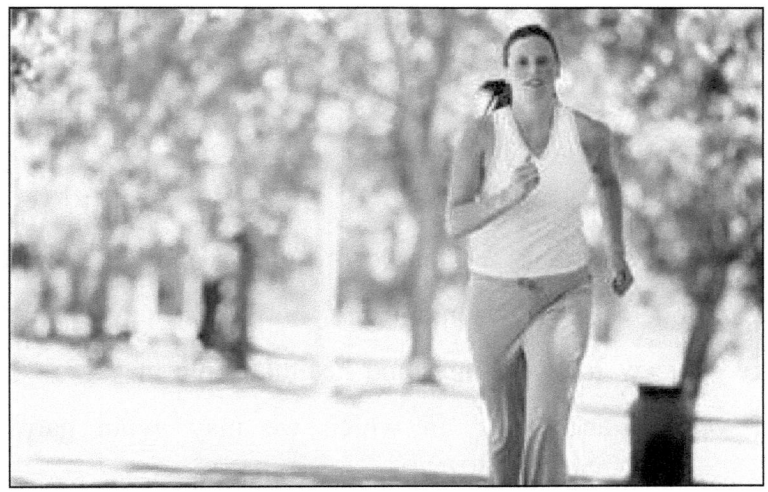

CHAPTER 4

SUPPLEMENTS AND OUR MINDSET

Synopsis

We have options, and that is to exercise and do our best to eat food that won't contaminate our bodies. We have to make choices to live longer and healthier. We may grow our own veggies and fruits, in which we may avoid harmful chemicals that will contaminate natural vitamins. Even more we might want to use some supplements.

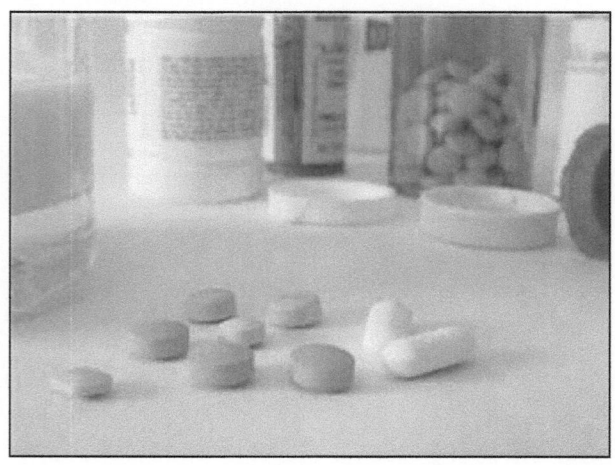

Purchasing

A healthier life has been helped by scientific measures, where new discoveries enlarge life span tremendously, as the measures taken reduce the risks of age-related suffering. The conditions often lead to major health problems and finally death, thus science is now working hard to find ways to live healthier while reducing aging.

What can I do personally to live longer?

Eat a balanced diet, exercise, learn about supplements continue doctor visits and seek out advice. Learn to listen and take action.

Let's look at some supplements BE SURE TO ALWAYS CHECK WITH YOUR DOCTOR FIRST!

HGH (Human Growth Hormone) is released by the pituitary gland. HGH is utilized in medicine to treat youngster's growth disorders and grownup growth hormone inadequacy. Reported effects on GH-deficient patients (but not on healthy individuals) include diminished body fat, expanded muscle mass, bone density, and energy levels, bettered skin tone/texture and immune system function.

In late years, growth hormone replacement therapies have become popular in the fight against aging and obesity.

We have aging hormones inside our body, which quit producing or secreting suitable elements that boost healthier living. Products with DHEA (Dehydroepiandrosterone) supercharge the immune system, which help in protecting us against disease.

A few small randomized clinical studies have discovered long-term supplementation of DHEA to better mood and alleviate depression or to lessen insulin resistance. Regular exercise is recognized to better DHEA production in the body. Some hypothesize that the growth in endogenous DHEA produced by calorie restriction is partly responsible for the longer life expectancy recognized to be associated with calorie restriction.

Ginkgo has evidenced to delay the process of aging while abbreviating health issues. It's an herbal extract, which promotes awareness and sounder brain functioning. In Germany physicians are utilizing Ginkgo products to treat patients enduring inadequate blood circulation, dementia, etc. The product works to enhance the brain's cells, by supplying natural nutrients.

Analyses are underway to prove that Ginkgo may better memory for those suffering from Alzheimer disease. Late studies demonstrated that those suffering from Alzheimer's displayed signs of remembering and communicating with other people more effectively than those taking other natural herbs. This herbal extract likewise has assisted those enduring PTSD and MPD

.While utilizing Ginkgo the only risks come from consuming the herb with feverfew, garlic, aspirin, ginger, MAO inhibitor, Coumadin or warfarin.

Flax-Seed Oil is a vegetable oil (polyunsaturated), which features ingredients like Omega-3, fatty acids, etc. Omega-3 has demonstrated evidence of depressing blood pressure, cholesterol, triglycerides, as well as cutting down sticky platelets.

Triglycerides are our bodies natural fats situated in tissues. Flax- Seed Oils may help to cut back strokes and heart attacks. Omega-3 was likewise found to better high-dense lipoproteins (HDLS), which is favorable cholesterol that helps the heart by decelerating clogging of arteries. Therefore, Omega-3 takes out LDL in the bloodstream for easier flow.

Flaxseed Oil has shown to slow or cut down development of tumors in the breast. Lignin is the responsible factor for reducing or treating cancers. Lignin is an estrogen founded compound. Chronic heart conditions are likewise reduced when you utilize flaxseed oils.

According to written reports, the only risk is that you may gain weight. Flaxseed oils are elevated in calories, and to lower the risks of weight gain you'd have to include flaxseed oils as a part of your daily caloric diet.

Melatonin is a hormone that releases through our pineal glands. It helps influence sleep and nerves. According to analyses, Melatonin increase may slow Alzheimer's, including dementia. It's likewise been discovered to retard tumor spreading, cancer and may retard the aging process.

When melatonin is low we may suffer stress, which induces nervous tension, constant worry, anxiety, panic attacks, trauma, and so forth. The downside is as we get older, we lose sound production of melatonin.

If you endure sleeping and nervous issues, Melatonin supplements may help relax your nerves and accomplish a restorative sleep. When you accomplish restorative rest, along with relaxation you'll find yourself feeling better daily. Compliment melatonin supplements with work outs and a balanced diet.

Visit your physician before beginning anything. Having an understanding of what your body needs is crucial for great health.

CHAPTER 5

EXERCISE AND CONCRETE TIPS

Synopsis

Exercise is crucial for all phases of life. It will make you feel younger, stronger and will help get the better of assorted diseases.

Slimming down is a process that takes time. Occasionally our perception on how to accomplish our weight loss goals keeps us from sticking with them leaving us defeated and with no success. To slim down and keep it off you have to adopt a fresh, healthy lifestyle that's both manageable and simple to stick with.

Below you'll find tips that can be used to melt pounds off and kept them off! There's no need to count calories, starve yourself, or cut back particular foods. By utilizing the method below you'll lose weight consistently and over time you'll reach your ideal weight.

Great Advice

As you grow old, exercises will take on a much more critical role, particularly in weight loss and establishing muscle mass. Exercise won't only assist you in slimming down, but it will likewise help you in keeping the weight off. Late studies show that ladies who continue to exercise on a regular basis are more successful at repressing weight, than those who don't.

Among the most useful workouts is aerobics. Aerobics will help you burn fat around the abdomen, as well as assorted other areas of the body and prevent the many causes of ill health, while you burn calories.

You are able to exercise a few days at home every week and get the results you would visiting the gymnasium. It takes time so don't expect a miracle overnight. As you begin aerobics, in turn you are able to prevent disease associated with being overweight.

A lot of individuals believe they have to run 1 to 2 miles daily and do assorted additional exercises to preserve health. The thought will often frighten them right out of exercise. The recommendation is fifteen to twenty minutes each day, no matter the complexity or ease of movement. It will pay off eventually. Walking briskly for a quarter-hour is a great exercise routine, which will help you burn up calories, as well as move the whole body.

Analyses are demonstrating that integrating aerobics into your life-style and making it a physical activity, like walking briskly each day, leaf raking, etc. is an good structured exercise program, which may improve heart activity, the respiratory system, fitness, and will cut down assorted diseases. What is more, you'll burn body fat, as well as calories.

Now, if you step-up walking , say adequate to ½ hour daily, you are able to attain a healthier way of life. In the morning you may walk 15 minutes, and walk a different 15 minutes later in the day. Every step you take to move the muscles is a different step closer to living longer, healthier, and happier.

Housecleaning, gardening, and so on are all activities that will help you burn calories. Most individuals will postpone today what they may have done yesterday. Try to prevent procrastinating. It takes only a couple of minutes to clean a small house, and once you finish you'll reap the rewards.

Alter your mentality. Throw out your "goal weight." Rather than centering on the amount of weight you wish to lose, take that same energy and direct it toward having a healthier life. Center on how good you look on the "inside" rather than how good you look on the outside. Long-lived weight loss comes

39

about when your internal organs are clean, functioning properly, and are well taken care of. Make certain you "look good" on the inside.

Eat as "organically" as imaginable. A lot of the foods consumed these days are the precise reasons why most weight loss prayers go unrequited. Conventional foods are full of pesticides, chemicals, and hormones that go directly into our system. Think about it, if the beef you eat is cut from a cow that has been shot with hormones in order to make it grow faster and larger, it's inevitable that those hormones will have the same impact on you.

Add a fruit or veggie to each meal. Even if you're eating something truly unhealthy adding fruits and vegetables will help fill you up quicker and give you healthy nutrients that you don't commonly get. This helps your body "look great" inside and out.

Begin eating at home more. It takes at least thirty-five minutes to drive, order, pick-up and take home food from restaurants. So why not take those thirty-five minutes to fix the same meal at home? It's healthier as you control the ingredients and portion sizes and you're less prone to germs and other disgusting things that weirdo's do to people's food in public places.

Get physical each day for at least half-hour - 2 of those days ought to be low impact. It's simple. Walk to the grocery store rather than driving. Go outside to play with your kids for half-hour or go out dancing. Look at exercise as a part of life, not chore. It's merely the art of moving your body! Make it a way of life. Find a physical exercise plan that works for you and stick to it.

Eat when you're hungry. Not doing so will only make you pig out in the long run. Just make sure that when you eat you manage your portion sizes and "treat" yourself to something tasty every once in a while so you don't feel punished or deprived.

If you're not hungry do not eat! I know that sounds like horse sense, but you won't believe how much we do it. It's simple for us to "snack" even when we're not hungry. This action is pure sabotage to your weight loss goals. Avoid it at all costs.

Maintain a positive mentality about your current body. Stop yourself every time you think or say something negative about your weight, eating habits, and body. If you happen to trip up, counteract that negative thought or statement with a positive one (out loud). We have to love our current body in order to reach our goals.

WRAPPING UP

Instincts were presented to you at birth. Those instincts may guide you better than anything in the world. Think about this: Through the years individuals have told you that if you adhere to a specific diet program you are able to slim down. The truth is no diet plan in the world will work for most individuals, as they live to be somebody they're not.

Instincts may guide you to greater health, yet most individuals will brush aside natural instincts. For example, something told you not to go to the bar last night. Yet, you might go anyhow and wonder why you don't feel well the following day.

If you leave nature to take its course, you'll notice the correct path to follow. You have to build wisdom to take you where you wish to go. Wisdom is perceptions and intelligence. When you utilize wisdom to arrive at decisions you utilize good judgment, while forming incisive thoughts that help you to see clearly. Wisdom furthers common sense. You attain wisdom by knowledge, understanding, insight, and so forth. So get started today.

One final point...

Regardless what you've gone through thus far in your quest to slim down, believe right now that this is true.

The secret is to kick your cravings by keeping your body fulfilled. The best way to do this is to front load your calories by consuming a healthy and hearty breakfast that's packed with protein.

This will not only jump start your metabolism, which will turn your body into a fat-burning machine throughout the day, but it will likewise help you avoid those cravings that lead to foul eating habits.

Beginning your day with a healthy breakfast not only helps to boost your metabolism and keep you burning off calories throughout the day, but it kicks you into a favorable mindset that begins your day in the life of a "dieter" strong!

Here's why breakfast is critical. When you first wake up in the morning, your body is prepared to hunt for food! Your metabolism is all fired up and your levels of cortisol and adrenaline are at their greatest.

If you don't provide your body with the energy it requires right away, your brain triggers your body to go in search of a different fuel source. So, it steals power from muscle, destroying your precious and beautiful muscle tissue.

If that's not bad enough, when you eat again later, your body and brain, which are still in starving mode, store the energy you feed it in the form of fat! By consuming a big hearty breakfast, you give your body exactly what it requires when it requires it and slowly smashes that addictive cycle of craving.

As well, remember:

1. Thoughts are things.

2. Words have power.

3. Feelings, emotions, are the juice, the electricity that powers the creation of your desires.

4. Action, lined up with thoughts and words, have more power than just pushing ahead without first putting thoughts, words and feelings in line ahead of those actions.

I hope .this book has given you a great starting point in your weight loss endeavor.

Printed by Libri Plureos GmbH in Hamburg,
Germany